NEATGEEK
Designs

How to use this planner?

The *'Get into Medical School'* Planner is a comprehensive guide designed for concise note-taking, collection of thoughts and medical application guidance.

There are three main sections of this planner which you will cover over the course of your application cycle:

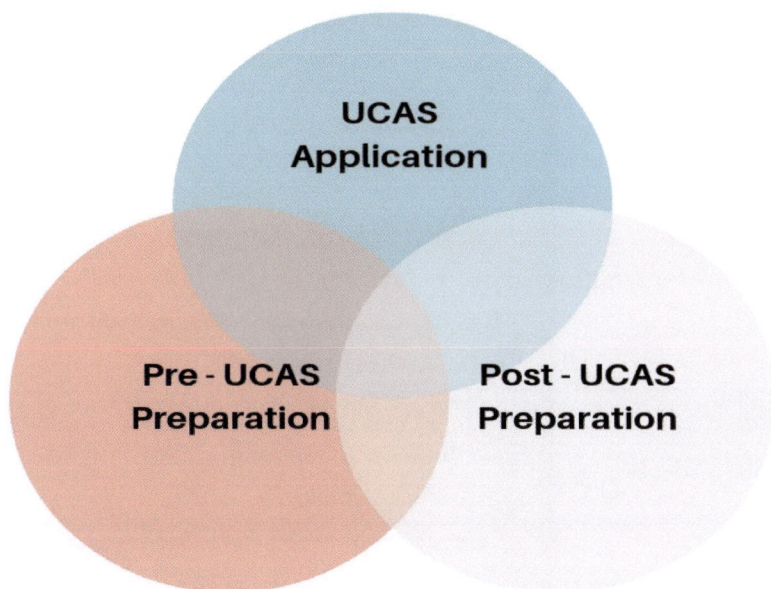

UCAS Application

Pre - UCAS Preparation

Post - UCAS Preparation

The workbook is designed such that the user 'fills in' the relevant information.
The mind-map and Interview answer guides should be written in concise bullet-point format, the idea being that (for interview purposes) it is most effective to understand concepts and ideas as opposed to memorising fully constructed answers.
You can use this workbook alongside other application literature to supplement your knowledge.

TIMELINE

My Checklist

Pre - UCAS Preparation

May

Jun

Jul

- Work Experience completed?
- Secured Predicted Grades (AAA)?
- UKCAT Test day booked?

UCAS Application

Aug

Sep

Oct

Nov

- UKCAT test completed?
- Personal Statement completed?
- Reference completed?
- UCAS Application sent off?

Post - UCAS Preparation

Dec

Jan

Feb

Mar

- Interview Preparation
- Offer holders days
- Securing the grades

WORK EXPERIENCE JOURNAL

Date :

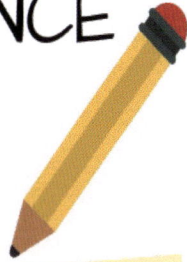

MY EXPERIENCE

What I saw :

What I learned from this :

I **WAS** surprised by :

I **WAS NOT** surprised by :

WORK EXPERIENCE JOURNAL

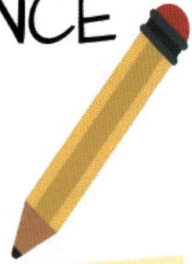

Date :

MY EXPERIENCE

What I saw :

What I learned from this :

I **WAS** surprised by :

I **WAS NOT** surprised by :

WORK EXPERIENCE JOURNAL

Date :

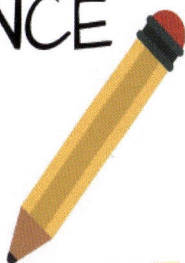

MY EXPERIENCE

What I saw :

What I learned from this :

I **WAS** surprised by :

I **WAS NOT** surprised by :

WORK EXPERIENCE JOURNAL

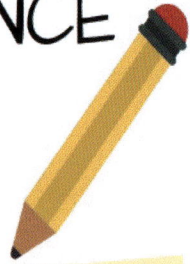

Date :

MY EXPERIENCE

What I saw :

What I learned from this :

I **WAS** surprised by :

I **WAS NOT** surprised by :

WORK EXPERIENCE JOURNAL

Date :

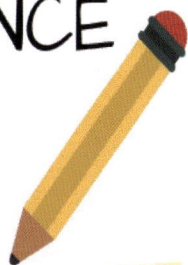

MY EXPERIENCE

What I saw :

What I learned from this :

I WAS surprised by :

I WAS NOT surprised by :

WORK EXPERIENCE JOURNAL

Date :

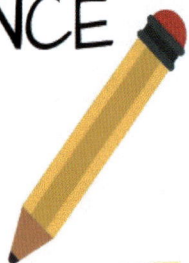

MY EXPERIENCE

What I saw :

What I learned from this :

I **WAS** surprised by :

I **WAS NOT** surprised by :

WORK EXPERIENCE JOURNAL

Date :

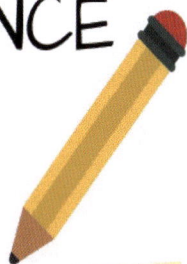

MY EXPERIENCE

What I saw :

What I learned from this :

I **WAS** surprised by :

I **WAS NOT** surprised by :

WORK EXPERIENCE JOURNAL

Date :

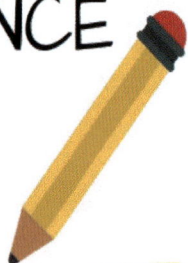

MY EXPERIENCE

What I saw :

What I learned from this :

I WAS surprised by :

I WAS NOT surprised by :

Pre - UCAS Preparation

What Is The UKCAT?

The UK Clinical Aptitude test is an admissions exam required by a number of UK Medical and Dental schools. The test is designed to assess the attributes and skills of applicants over each annual admissions cycle. Familiarise yourself with the format of the test by visiting: **UKCAT Official Website © at www.ucat.ac.uk.**

The 2019 test consists of five main topics:

Verbal Reasoning

Decision making

Quantitative Reasoning

Abstract Reasoning

Situational Judgement

Why do you need a Strategy for the UKCAT?

'You can't revise for the UKCAT!'

You've probably heard this phrase from your peers and many past applicants.
The statement is partly correct; the UKCAT is not a traditional exam.
It's not theory based – the test is based on your ability to apply different skillsets.
However, just like a marathon runner trains for a race, anyone can prepare for the UKCAT.

The strategy used by most students is *'Practice Makes Perfect!'* Whilst this strategy is effective, if you do not know how to approach each section of the test correctly - no amount of practice will get you an amazing score.

The 'How to sail through the UKCAT Tip sheet' is a *no-waffle, straight-to-the-point* guide on how to tackle the UKCAT. These are simple tips that every applicant should know, but year-after-year applicants trip up on the same mistakes.

When should I start revising for the UKCAT?

There is no set start date for UKCAT revision, but it is recommended that you begin familiarising yourself with the topics at least 6 weeks prior to test day. Remember, training for the UKCAT is like training for a race – you won't ace it overnight. Consistency and practice (the right type of practice – that is) are key.

There are several non-intensive UKCAT training strategies that you can adopt prior to test day, including: reading newspaper articles everyday (building verbal reasoning skills), practicing mental maths and sudoku (building quantitative reasoning alongside abstract reasoning). There are several resources you can use to prepare for the UKCAT – a number of them are discussed in this Tip Sheet!

VERRBAL REASONING

The verbal reasoning section assesses your ability to critically evaluate information presented in a written form. You'll have 21 minutes to answer 44 questions. That gives you just over 1 minute to read, comprehend and answer questions on each short piece of text.

The verbal reasoning section is a challenge for students who do not recognise, and actively avoid, the common pitfalls.

Here are three important tips for 'SAILING THROUGH' the verbal reasoning section:

1. **Read the question first:**

   Do not read the excerpt first - you simply do not have enough time.
   Always read the question first
   This method allows you to rapidly identify keywords that will help you navigate the text more effectively.

2. **Focus on the keywords:**

   What keywords appear in the question?
   Do these words also occur in the text?
   Scan the text for the keywords.
   Only read the sentences encompassing your keyword.
   Do these sentences include your answer?
   If not - search for the most likely option, given the context of the text.

3. **If all else fails, GUESS.**

   The applicants who tend to do best on the UKCAT are those applicants that recognise that they simply do not have the time to answer every question.

   If it comes to guessing, go with the 'educated' guess. Remember, you can always go back to a question if you have time at the end of each section.

Attempt the Verbal Reasoning Activity on the next page, applying this strategy

Verbal Reasoning Activity

Change is an inescapable facet of all life. The very fact that our souls, like transient globes of light, must one day flicker to nonexistence, actuates this argument for change. Most people of today's world may be delivered and die in the very same town, never having experienced another vicinity, or leading a wholly fulfilled life. The argument for change cannot suffice in such cases. Nevertheless, I, in my short 17 years of life, have lived through a few drastic changes, and today will be a new one. The first 'drastic' change that I ever experienced was when my family relocated from England to the state of India in 2085, I was only seven years old and had never travelled by air, but had only read of it in the tales of old, when humans had endless supplies of fossil fuels and dealt with them carelessly. I expect that in those days, men and women may have travelled by air at least once a year, as annual holiday.

(1) Most people in today's world do not lead a fulfilled life

- (a) True
- (b) False
- (c) Can't Tell

(2) How old is the author?

- (a) 7
- (b) 10
- (c) 24
- (d) 17

(3) Tales of old describe humans as:

- (a) Dealing with fossil fuels carelessly
- (b) Never travelling by air
- (c) Taking an annual holiday more than once a year
- (d) Never taking an annual holiday

(4) When does the author expect to experience a drastic change?

    (a) In 2085

    (b) Never

    (c) Today

    (d) Tomorrow

DECISION MAKING

In this section of the test, you will have 31 minutes to answer 29 questions. You will be assessed on your ability to make sound decisions and judgements using complex information.

There are two essential tips for _'SAILING THROUGH'_ this section of the test:

(1) Take your time to UNDERSTAND the question:

As this section of the test is about understanding relationships and information, do not rush a question unless you know that solving the question will take too long. In which case, select a feasible answer and move on.

(2) Make use of your whiteboard

There are several reasons why students deliberately avoid using the whiteboard. Some feel that writing down their 'working out' is time consuming. However, students who make use of the whiteboard tend to get more done in less time. Writing the key elements of the scenario will help you establish logic and reason. Venn diagrams are becoming increasingly popular UKCAT questions – so read up on these. Remember, the answer is right there in the options. If in doubt... guess. You have a 1 in 4 chance of guessing right!

Decision Making Activity

Of all the UKCAT applicants in the last 10 years, none of them made use of their whiteboards

(a) Only applicants who used their whiteboards applied to the UKCAT in the last 10 years

(b) UKCAT applicants never use their whiteboards

(c) Some UKCAT applicants have used their whiteboards in the last 10 years

(d) 10 years ago, UKCAT applicants used their whiteboards more

(e) Of all the whiteboard users in the last 10 years, none of them where UKCAT applicants

QUANTITATIVE REASONING

You'll need to answer 24 mathematical questions in 36 minutes time. This section of the test calls for critical evaluation of information presented in numerical form.

Here are three essential tips for 'SAILING THROUGH' this section of the test:

(1) Learn the keyboard shortcuts when operating the virtual calculator

This is a huge time – saver!
Head over to the official UKCAT website and learn how to operate the virtual calculator, including the keyboard shortcuts. Minimise time wasted clicking the calculator buttons and you WILL see an improvement in your overall performance.

(2) Boost your Mental Maths!

Daily practice of simple mental maths (e.g. multiplication, unit conversions), even as late as one week prior to test day has been shown to improve performance in the quantitative reasoning test.
Practice converting percentages and decimals in your head.
Be familiar with unit conversions.
Knowing the basics goes a long way in the test!

(3) Practice!

You don't need to be a Maths-wiz to score high in this section of the test.
But you will need to practice, practice, practice.
There are a number of online mental maths resources and a huge bank of questions on the UKCAT official website.

Cheatbox: What to Practice?

Before test day, be sure to brush up on GCSE Maths. You don't need to spend a huge amount of time on this – but going over a select group of popular UKCAT topics will undoubtably strengthen your maths skills and boost your confidence. **GCSE BBC Bitesize ©** is a brilliant resource!

These topics below recur yearly in the UKCAT question bank

Basic Arithmetic

Proportionality

Percentage, fractions and changes

Ratios

Speed, Distance and Time

Money, Tax & Exchanges

Geometry

Population densities

Averages and ranges

Time

Rates

Quantitative Reasoning Activity

The Ladies Gym	
Package	**Price (£)**
3-month Membership	180
Basic Package (1 year)	240
Standard Membership (1 year)	275
Premium Membership (1 year)	360

The Ladies Gym always sells twice as many 'Basic Packages' compared to '3-month membership'

(1) On Monday, the gym made £960 selling Basic Packages, how many 3-month membership packages where sold?

(a) 1
(b) 4
(c) 3
(d) 2

(2) How much more expensive is the price of the 'Standard Membership' compared to the 'Basic Package'?

(a) + 14.6%
(b) + 14.7%
(c) + 14.5 %
(d) + 13.8 %
(e) + 13.9 %

(3) Susan renews her 3-month membership each time it runs out. How much money would Susan have saved last year if she'd opted to purchase a Standard Membership (1 year).

(a) 425
(b) 435
(c) 445
(d) 455

(4) Only 15% of gym members purchase the premium membership, if 164 members joined last year, how many of them are premium members?

(a) 27
(b) 25
(c) 29
(d) 26

(5) How much money does a Premium gym member spend weekly (assuming 52 weeks in a year)?

    (a) £9

    (b) £20

    (c) £15

    (d) £7

    (e) £6

ABSTRACT REASONING

You'll be given 13 minutes to answer 55 **'Abstract Reasoning'** questions.

Some people are naturally inclined to spotting abstract trends and patterns, but this doesn't mean that the skill cannot be learned. In fact, Abstract reasoning is the section of the test that candidates are most likely to show significant improvement, with just a little practice.

Here are three essential tips for 'SAILING THROUGH' this section of the test:

(1) **Know what to look for**

Knowing what to look for only comes through practice: **Get into Medical School - 600 UKCAT Practice Questions** © *is a fantastic resource*

Commonly Tested:

- Position
- Rotation and Orientation
- Symmetry
- Colour
- Order
- Numbers
- Angles
- Intersections
- Reflection
- Curved sides/straight sides

(2) Investigate the simplest box first:

- What do all the members of **SET A/B** have in common?
- Are distractors present?

There is no strict guide on how to spot the pattern.

However, a good way to start is by looking at the simplest box (of a set) first.

For example, if the simplest box has 1 black square – a common element could be colour (black) or the presence of a square (shape).

Explore all themes, applying trial and error.

Be quick about it - If you perceive that rotation is not a common theme, then move on to symmetry. If symmetry fails, investigate use of angles … and so on.

Your method will be different to everybody else's – Find one that works for you.

(3) Go with your instinct:

The old saying *'you know, when you know'* truly does apply here.

Your brain can pick up visual information in patterns before you've had time to consciously rationalise it.

You may instinctively feel that a particular image goes with a particular set - or perhaps it belongs to neither set.

If you feel this inclination - go with it.

You can always change your answer if you have time at the end.

Abstract Reasoning Activity

Determine whether 1-4 belong to set A (A), set B (B) or Neither (C)

Set A

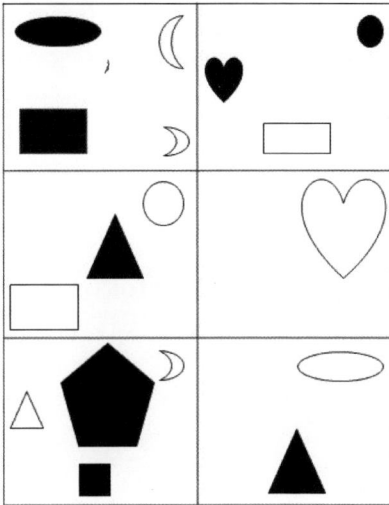

Set B

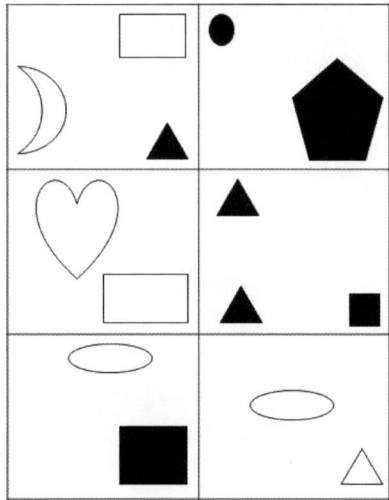

1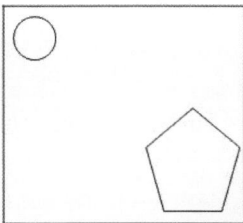

2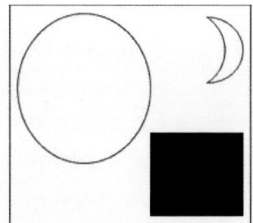

3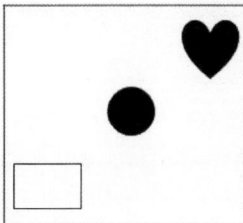

4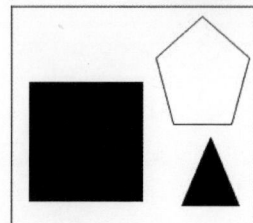

SITUATIONAL JUDGEMENT

Your ability to understand real world situations will be assessed in the Situational Judgement Test (SJT).

You'll be given a number of scenarios and asked to select a solution that best resolves the presented problem.

Remember that Justice, Autonomy, Beneficence Non-maleficence are key attributes.

The test will select for candidates whose ideologies best represent these attributes.

Here are three essential tips for *'SAILING THROUGH'* the Situational Judgment test:

1. **Remember what it means to be a GOOD Doctor or Dentist**

   When answering questions, put yourself in the shoes of a health-care professional.
   How would you expect your doctor to act?
   You'd probably expect your Doctor or Dentist to be honest and have integrity.
   Keep in mind these themes when answering the questions.

2. **Choose the MOST appropriate response**

   Sometimes it's a lose-lose situation, this test judges your ability to select the lesser evil.
   What option, in the long-run, will prove to be the lesser evil?

3. **Read up on GMC/GDC guidelines**

   You should know how Doctors and Dentists are expected to behave, as implemented by their relevant regulating bodies (General Medical / Dental Councils)

If a practicing doctor/ dentist or student goes against these guidelines, how are colleges expected to react?

It is worthwhile reading up on the guidelines as they shed light on appropriate responses.

9 out of 10 times, the SJT questions are based on handling situations where a professional or student has gone against the regulations.

Cheatbox: Useful Resources

Good Medical Practice (For Doctors): *www.gmc-uk.org/ethical-guidance*
Standards and Guidance for Dental Practice: *www.gdc-uk.org/professionals/standards*

Remember, all SJT scenarios boil down to three principles:

Autonomy
Beneficence and Non-maleficence
Justice

Sarah is a first-year medical student. She is shadowing a local GP, Dr. Kaur, and notices that Dr. Kaur is persistently rude to the practice nurse, Beatrice. When Dr. Kaur leaves, Sarah overhears Beatrice talking to the practice receptionist. Beatrice says that Dr. Kaur's attitude is beginning to make her feel uncomfortable and patients are also picking up on it.

Rate the appropriateness of Sarah's response:

(1) Do nothing

- (a) Appropriate
- (b) Appropriate but not ideal
- (c) Inappropriate
- (d) Very Inappropriate

(2) File a complaint against Dr. Kaur

- (a) Appropriate
- (b) Appropriate but not ideal
- (c) Inappropriate
- (d) Very Inappropriate

(3) Suggest to Dr. Kaur that he ought to treat Beatrice with more respect

- (a) Appropriate
- (b) Appropriate but not ideal
- (c) Inappropriate
- (d) Very Inappropriate

(4) Discuss the matter with your supervisor at university and seek further advice.

- (a) Appropriate
- (b) Appropriate but not ideal
- (c) Inappropriate
- (d) Very Inappropriate

(5) Comfort Beatrice and tell her to ignore Dr. Kaur's attitude

- (a) Appropriate
- (b) Appropriate but not ideal
- (c) Inappropriate
- (d) Very Inappropriate

TEST DAY TIPS

1. Eat a Good Breakfast

You may have spent the entire summer practicing, or maybe you just practiced a week before test day.
It all boils down to how you perform on the day!
So, may sure that you start the day off with a GOOD breakfast.

2. Be Decisive

The worst thing you can be on test-day is indecisive.
Remember, you either know the answer or you don't.
If you know the answer – brilliant!
If you don't, take an educated guess.
The test is not negatively marked.
You won't lose points by selecting the wrong answer.
In fact, you're likely to get at least 1 out of 4 guesses right – that's 25%

3. So, you didn't get the score you wanted?

Remember that the UKCAT is only one element of an otherwise complex admissions process.
Your personal statement, grades and reference all come into play.
Universities will look at each candidate holistically.
So, don't feel dismayed if you do not get the score you wanted.
Pick yourself up and focus on strengthening the rest of your application!

Familiarise yourself with UKCAT questions using:

- **UKCAT Official question bank ©**
- *600 UKCAT Practice Questions ©*
- **Medify UKCAT Practice ©**

MY PROFILE

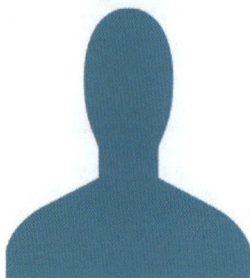

My **GCSE** Results:

My Predicted/ Attained **A-LEVEL** Results:

I scored .... in the UK Clinical Aptitude Test (UKCAT)

Do my qualifications meet the requirements?   **Yes / NO**

MY PROFILE

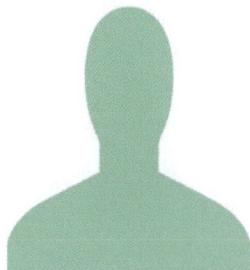

My **Strengths** :

My **Weaknesses:**

I am **suited** to Medicine because:

MEDICAL SCHOOLS

My **1st** UCAS Choice:

Entry **Requirements** are:

Advantages :

Drawbacks :

MY RESEARCH

This Medical School is famous for :

Current Developments at this Medical School :

MEDICAL SCHOOLS

My **2nd** UCAS Choice:

Entry **Requirements** are:

Advantages :

Drawbacks :

MY RESEARCH

This Medical School is famous for :

Current Developments at this Medical School :

MEDICAL SCHOOLS

My **3rd** UCAS Choice:

Entry **Requirements** are:

Advantages :

Drawbacks :

MY RESEARCH

This Medical School is famous for :

Current Developments at this Medical School :

MEDICAL SCHOOLS

My **4th** UCAS Choice:

Entry **Requirements** are:

Advantages :

Drawbacks :

MY RESEARCH

This Medical School is famous for :

Current Developments at this Medical School :

PLANNING

WORK EXPERIENCE

GOALS AND AMBITIONS

★ ....

★ ....

★ ....

PERSONAL STATEMENT

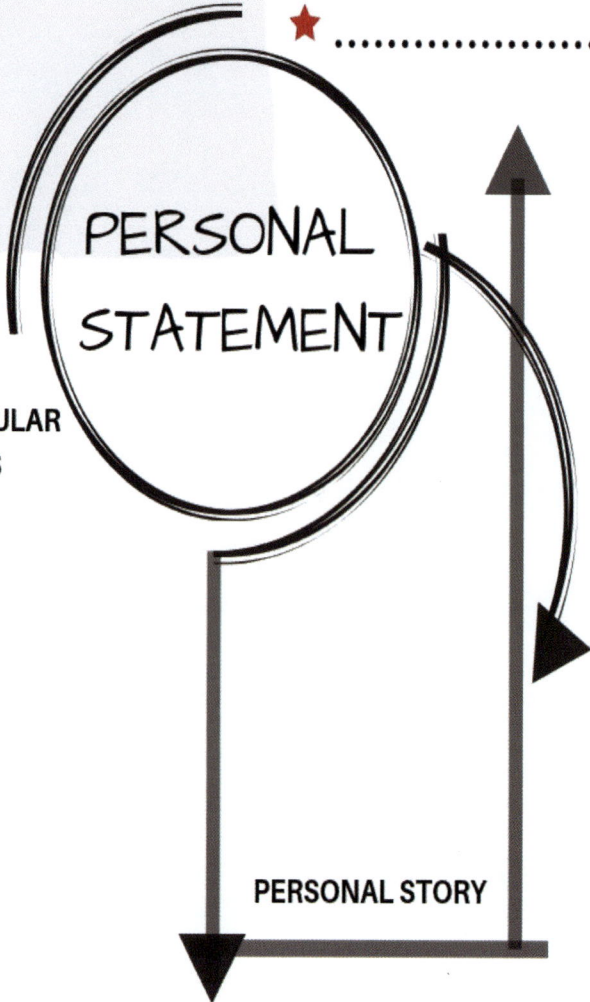

EXTRA CURRICULAR ACTVITIES

PERSONAL STORY

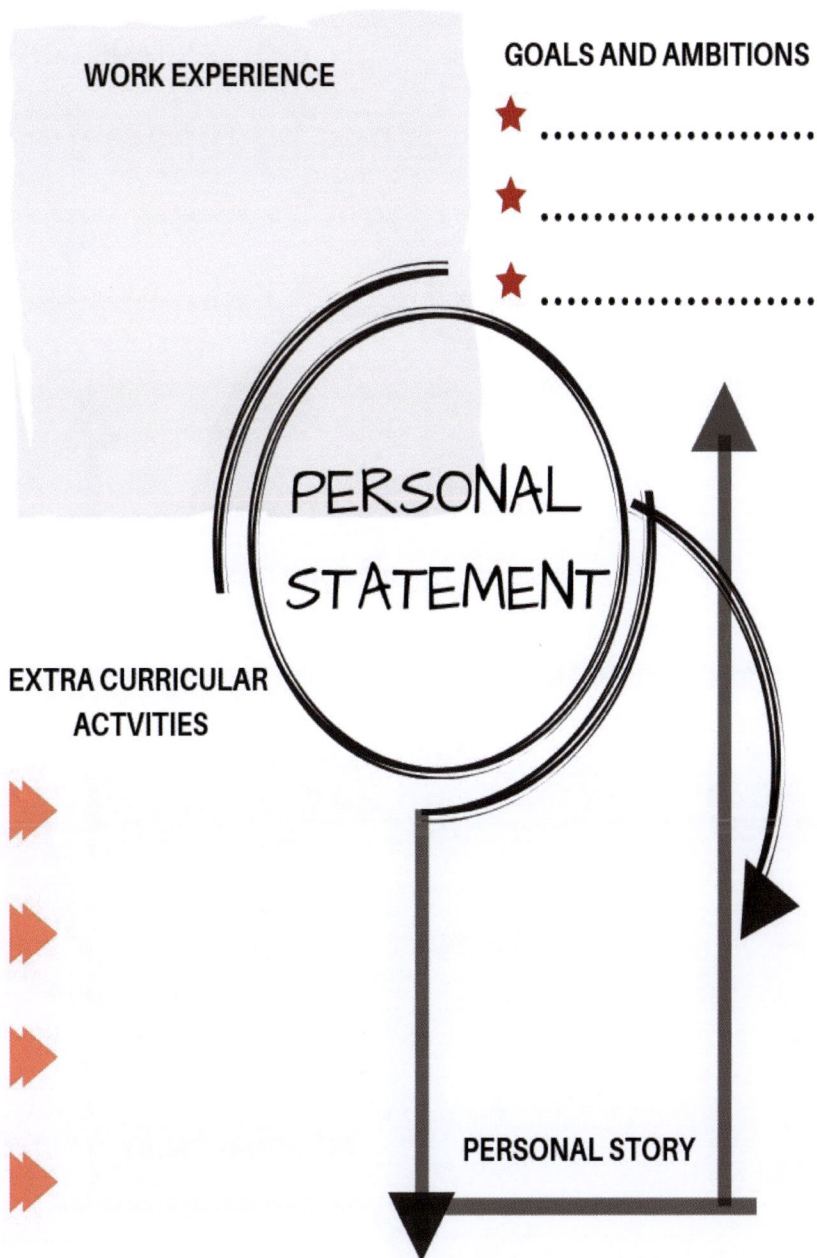

PLANNING

WORK EXPERIENCE

GOALS AND AMBITIONS

★ ....

★ ....

★ ....

PERSONAL

STATEMENT

**EXTRA CURRICULAR
ACTVITIES**

PERSONAL STORY

PLANNING

WORK EXPERIENCE

GOALS AND AMBITIONS

★ ....

★ ....

★ ....

PERSONAL STATEMENT

EXTRA CURRICULAR ACTVITIES

PERSONAL STORY

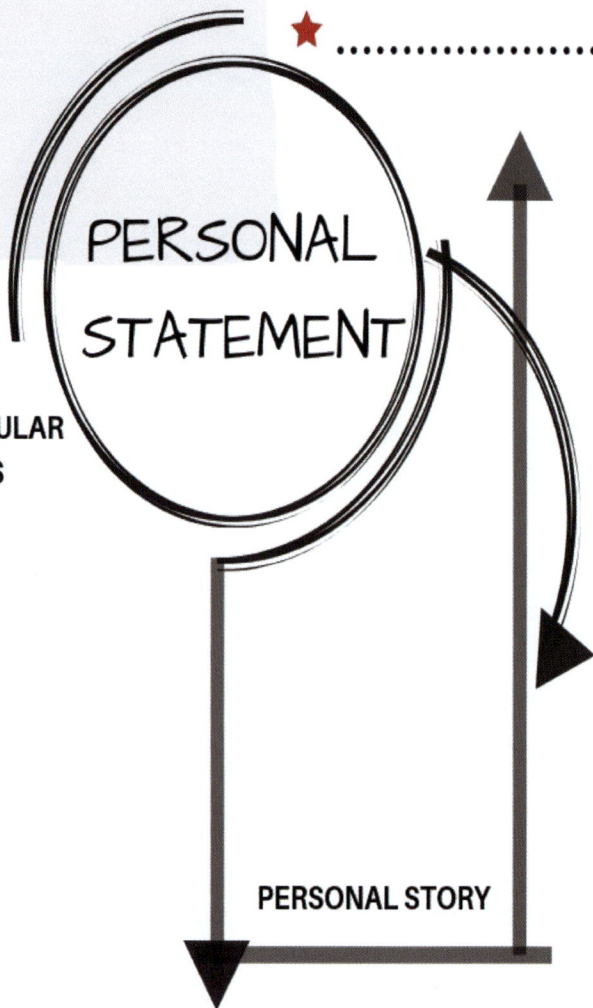

PLANNING

WORK EXPERIENCE

GOALS AND AMBITIONS

★ ....

★ ....

★ ....

PERSONAL STATEMENT

EXTRA CURRICULAR ACTVITIES

PERSONAL STORY

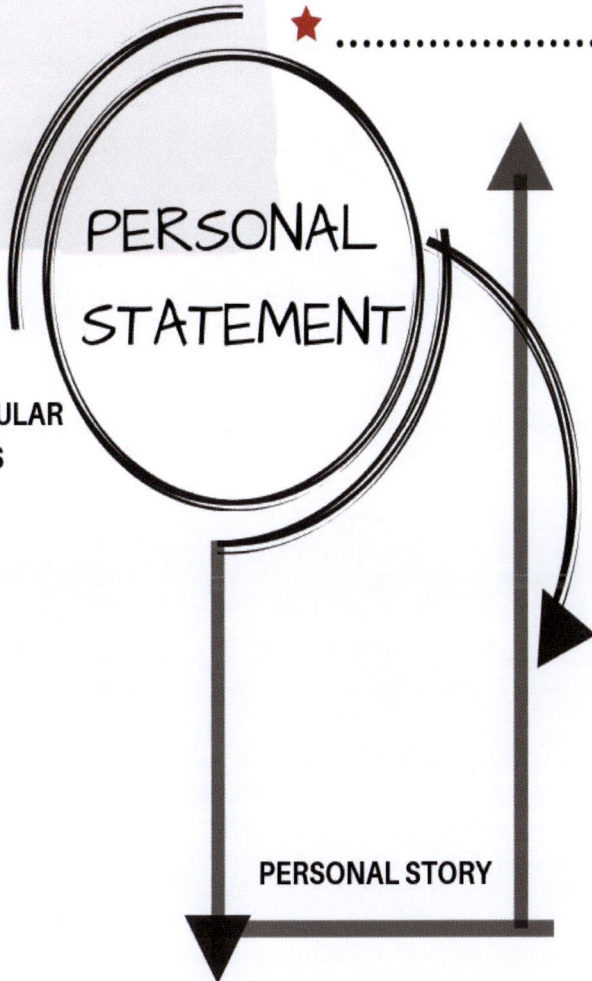

PLANNING

Personal Story

Add a personal touch to your statement
Has Medicine contributed to you, or a
family member significantly?

PERSONAL
STATEMENT

Be Descriptive:

How did this personal experience affect you?
What has this taught you about yourself?
Remember ... don't lie!

PLANNING

WORK EXPERIENCE

Describe something you saw whilst
on work shadowing , that you'd like to
include in your personal statement ...

PERSONAL
STATEMENT

Be Descriptive:

What did you learn?
Why did this surprise you?
Or, why did this not surprise you?
What did this experience teach you about Medicine?

PLANNING

EXTRACURRICULAR ACTIVTIES

Describe what you do in your free time.
Why is making time for yourself important?
Will your hobby make you a better Doctor?

PERSONAL STATEMENT

Be Descriptive:

When did you start this hobby?
What has this hobby taught you?
Remember ... don't lie!

PLANNING

GOALS AND AMBITIONS

Describe your goals and ambitions:
What are you driven by?
Where do you see yourself in 10 years time?

PERSONAL
STATEMENT

Be Descriptive:

What attracts you most about medicine?
If you like to help people, back up your claims with examples?
Why is studying medicine important to you?
How will you contribute to the medical school?

BACKGROUND
INFORMATION

What are the issues surrounding the NHS?

What recent medical news have you recently come across?

What difficulties are posed for GPs?

Where do you think the NHS should allocate funds?

BACKGROUND
INFORMATION

Why is stem cell research important?

Why has There been a rise in the measles epidemic?

Why are genetic disorders difficult to treat?

What is gene therapy?

ABOUT THE MEDICAL SCHOOL

What interests you about our curriculum?

Why have you chosen our medical school?

Do you know about small group learning?

What are the advantages and disadvantages of problem based learning?

ABOUT STUDYING MEDICINE

Do you have the ability to be a doctor? If so, why?

What branch of medicine would interest you, and why?

Why did you apply to Medicine rather than Nursing?

What is the most important medical advance in the last century?

ABOUT STUDYING MEDICINE

Discuss a key historical figure that you think has contributed to Medicine.

What is the greatest public health advance in the 20th century?

Has social media impacted Medicine?

Have developments in IT influenced Medicine?

ABOUT YOU

Why do you want to study medicine?

What did you learn from your work experience?

Why are good communication skills essential?

How do you handle stress?

INTERPERSONAL SKILLS

Have you ever been in a team? - What was your contribution?

Discuss a situation where you've had to solve a team problem

How do you cope with criticism?

What are your hobbies?

What are your personal shortcomings?

MEDICINE & SOCIETY

How do politics affect health care?

What are the government priorities in health care?

What is meant by `Inequalities in health' ?

· What is holistic medicine and is it within the NHS remit?

MEDICINE & SOCIETY

What is the greatest threat to the UK population's health?

What are the arguments for and against banning tobacco?

Should doctors be able to turn off life support systems?

Discuss your experience of a multi cultural environment.

WORK EXPERIENCE

What surprised you during your work experience?

What key things did you learn from work experience?

Is work/life balance important?

Did you see anything you didn't like during work experience?

MY REFLECTIONS

Post-UCAS Preparation: **Notes**

MY REFLECTIONS

Post-UCAS Preparation: **Notes**

MY REFLECTIONS

MY REFLECTIONS

MY REFLECTIONS

MY REFLECTIONS

Post-UCAS Preparation: **Notes**

MY REFLECTIONS

MY REFLECTIONS

MY REFLECTIONS

MY REFLECTIONS

UKCAT ANSWERS

VERBAL REASONING ANSWERS

(1) A

Keywords to look for: **'Fulfilled Life'**

'Most people of today's world may be delivered and die in the very same town, never having experienced another vicinity, or leading a wholly fulfilled life.'

(2) D

This question is asking about numbers – where is age talked about in the text?

'I, in my short 17 years of life'

(3) A

Keywords to look for: **'Tales of old'**

'…in the tales of old, when humans had endless supplies of fossil fuels and dealt with them carelessly.'

(4) C

Keywords to look for: *'drastic change'*

'Nevertheless, I, in my short 17 years of life, have lived through a few drastic changes, and today will be a new one'

Did you spot the keywords?

DESCISION MAKING ANSWERS

Answer: E

This is a simple test of logic.
The information in the statement tells you that no UKCAT applicants in the last 10 years used their whiteboard.
Select the option that aligns with this scenario – the answer is E

QUANTITATIVE REASONING ANSWERS

(1) D

'The Ladies Gym always sells twice as many 'Basic Packages' compared to '3-month membership'

The price of the Basic Package is £240.

Working:

- 960 ÷ 240 = 4
- 4 ÷ 2 = 2

(2) A

Calculate percentage difference

Working: $\frac{275-240}{240} \times 100 = 14.58$

- Did you round up?
- Did you get a percentage increase or decrease?

(3) C

'Susan renews her 3-month membership each time it runs out' – This means Sarah renews 4 times a year.

Working:

- 180 × 4 = 720
- 720 – 275 = 445

(4) B

Working:

- $0.15 \times 164 = 24.6$
- Did you round up?

(5) D

Working:

- $360 \div 52 = 6.92$
- Did you round up?

ABSTRACT REASONING ANSWERS

Set A: A shape with a curved edge is always in the UPPER right corner
Set B: A shape with straight edges is always in the LOWER right corner
Look out for distractors!

- (1) B
- (2) C
- (3) A
- (4) B

SITUATIONAL JUDGEMENT ANSWERS

Note that this question is assessing your ability to measure appropriateness in a real-life scenario. As a medical student, you may very well find yourself in this particular scenario, as you'll spend plenty time shadowing doctors.

(1) D

Doing nothing is a very inappropriate response. By neglecting the situation and not addressing the issue you are inadvertently allowing it to propagate. If Dr. Kaur's attitude is affecting staff and patients, it needs to be addressed.

(2) D

Filing a complaint against a member of staff without making them aware of the issue at hand is always inappropriate. This should be a last resort.

(3) B

Sarah is not highlighting the problem – only giving a suggestion. Dr. Kaur may treat Beatrice better following this advice, but what about his treatment of other staff?

(4) A

Sarah is a first-year medical student. Seeking out advice from the university is always the BEST call!

(5) D

Telling Beatrice to ignore Dr. Kaur's attitude not only dismisses Beatrice's right to express herself, but also does not bring awareness to the issue.

Printed in Great Britain
by Amazon